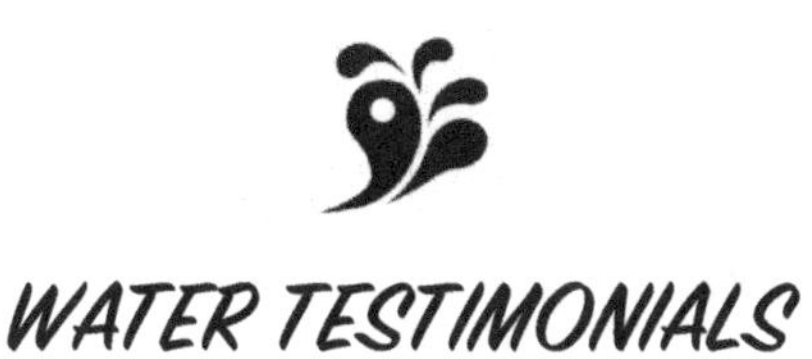

WATER TESTIMONIALS

"I met Jodi several years ago. While athletic, I'd never worked with a personal trainer, much less been in a gym environment. I needed professional training with balance issues, strength training for my lower back, and also needed to drop a few pounds to lower some critical blood levels (cholesterol and glucose). Mission accomplished thanks to her great skill as a trainer.

My husband took up water aerobics, along with me, during the hot summer months in Arizona. Several year ago he had serious back surgery which affected his lower back strength and mobility. Jodi focused on personalized training with him. For him, it was a wonderful experience with a great outcome!

Jodi approaches her training in a 'big picture' manner. Personal well-being, fitness, nutrition, and follow-up. Both of us are healthier because of her expertise. Without a doubt, a true pro, she takes great pride in her profession and truly cares for each individual she trains. Thank you so much, Jodi, for your friendship and skill at training."

—**Kathy and Laird Anderson**

"As a physician, I regularly counsel my patients on the health benefits of exercise. More than any pill or fad, exercise reverses diabetes, depression, anxiety, heart disease, high blood pressure—and has been linked to lower rates of dementia, cancer, and back pain. I was not prepared, however, for the profound impact Jodi's program would have on my health, personally. As I followed her program, I watched my physical and mental health improve dramatically. I cannot recall a time when I've felt better. Her program is unique because it builds strength and endurance, along with supporting the health of joints, lymphatics, skin, flexibility, and balance. Trust her and let her do her job using her more than thirty years of training and teaching. Your only regret will be not starting earlier."

—**Maggie Williams, MD Diplomat, American Board of Family Medicine**

"I have been an on and off exerciser for many years, but I haven't found an exercise program I enjoy or look forward to as much as working out with Jodi. She uses a holistic approach to exercise—her workouts challenge you and push your limits and, at the same time, she creates an environment in which you want to work hard and you feel encouraged and supported. As the weather warmed up, Jodi moved our workouts into the pool and these pool workouts have been a godsend over the hot Arizona summers. It is challenging to maintain a regular exercise program in the extreme heat of an Arizona summer, but Jodi has found a way to provide her clients with consistent, challenging, and effective exercise with her water exercise program. I actually think my body and muscle tone has changed more significantly working out in the pool than it has doing any other consistent exercise. Using the natural resistance of the water along with her many tricks and tools to make the workouts more challenging, Jodi has created exercise that targets all your muscles and also leaves you feeling great!"

—**Rachel Boyer Shuman**

WATER EXERCISE

For Exercise Enthusiasts,
Teachers/Trainers,
and Health Support

WATER EXERCISE

For Exercise Enthusiasts,
Teachers/Trainers,
and Health Support

By Jodi Stokes, BS Exercise Science

Published by Jodi Books-Stokes
Scottsdale, AZ
www.jodistokes.com

DEDICATION

In loving memory of my father, who was disciplined in his exercise beliefs and never took his health for granted. He gave me my work ethic, his constant support, and a reason to do what I do for a living.

TABLE OF CONTENTS

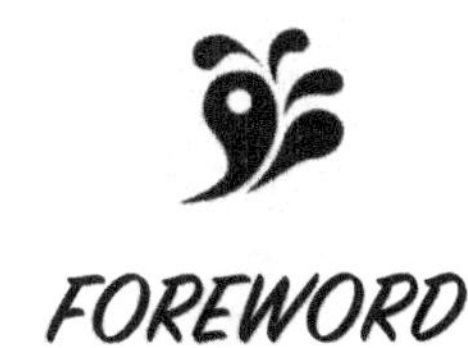

FOREWORD

My story begins during spring break of 2001 with my sons in tow. I was traveling from California to my home town of Scottsdale Arizona. The boys were small at the time, so it was easy to please them with simple and enjoyable things to do on spring break, such as visiting my parents. The trip had a special purpose, however, to help my dad work out in the water to assist with his post-polio syndrome. His symptoms included: falling frequently, muscle atrophy, progressive muscle and joint weakness, pain, and general fatigue.

Make no mistake, although the man was born with a crippling disease, you would have never known! He *never* parked in handicapped spaces, he rode his bike, swam, and did fifty push-ups and sit-ups every night. Dad took cod liver oil before we all knew it was an Omega-3. So, when I looked at my dad, I never thought of him with a physical limitation. I looked up to him and admired him for his strength and fortitude. However, at that time he had been experiencing progressive degenerative symptoms of his disease.

The first morning of that spring break, I took Dad out to the pool for his first lesson. Being degreed and with fifteen years of health and physical training experience under my belt at the time, I was able to design some very intricate lesson plans and workout diagrams which looked like stick figures with water waves drawn through them. Pretty ingenious? Well, Dad thought so anyway. He had them perfectly laminated and put in a binder for our next session, so they would not get wet.

We worked up to fifty-five minutes by the end of the week. My dad told me his range of motion had increased significantly and the buoyancy of the water enabled him to do more strength work than he was ever able to do on land.

With great sadness I must tell you Dad has since passed away. Twenty years later, though, I am finally pursuing this dream. I know he would have wanted me to finish this project to help others grow stronger or help with any physical limitation they may need to overcome. Because of him I have adopted the phrase, "Exercise is not a chore, it is a privilege."

Now, with thirty of more years of exercise experience, added certifications, awards, and having trained hundreds of clients… I am pleased to bring you *Water Exercise*.

—Jodi Books-Stokes

Jodi Books-Stokes

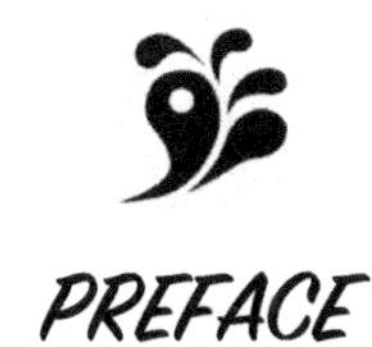

PREFACE

Water exercise is vastly becoming the wave of the future in workout programming with fitness enthusiasts. Research dictates that the buoyancy effect of the water eliminates shock and trauma to the joints and surrounding tissues. The hydrostatic pressure reduces swelling, and the cooling effect of the water keeps body temperature lower for a longer duration, which ultimately affects caloric expenditure. It is also believed the workload placed on the body can be twelve times greater in the water than on land, due to the constant resistance placed on the muscles, or double concentric contraction.

Water exercise benefits all types of needs ranging from pre-post-natal, injury prevention and recovery, arthritics, post-polio, and helps those who suffer from MS or other limitations that may prevent them from participating in "on land" exercise programs. It is also beneficial as a vehicle for seasoned athletes.

Water exercise will improve cardiovascular strength, muscular strength/ endurance, flexibility, range of motion, and balance. By focusing on the strong structural center referred to as the core, we are able to engage the stomach muscles for the duration of the exercises which, in turn, will strengthen the back.

The water pressure on the lungs encourages deeper breathing, improved lung capacity, and a more efficient cardiorespiratory system. Breathing during all phases of an exercise routine should be continuous and rhythmic.

Jodi Books-Stokes is currently certified in these programs, and has worked with these issues for more than twenty years.

ACKNOWLEDGMENTS

Special thanks to Mom! Also, a loving memory of a woman who came to all of my exercise classes. Who, though she never smoked, fought stage-four lung cancer for four years and still managed to take cycle and water classes.

And, thanks to my ever supportive students, clients, friends, and family. Because of their years of love and encouragement through all of my fitness endeavors, this project was accomplished.

THANK YOU, THANK YOU, THANK YOU, God and the Universe.

INTRODUCTION

When I received my bachelor of science in exercise science from the University of Arizona, I began my lifelong commitment to fitness/wellness at the world-renowned Canyon Ranch Spa, where I truly found my love for teaching water exercise. Soon after that, I designed the water program at the Hyatt Gainey Ranch and quickly became the fitness manager at the brand new Scottsdale Princess Resort and Spa.

After marrying and having two boys, I found myself whisked off to Valencia, California, for about seventeen years. Once there, my world and opportunity for expansion in the fitness industry grew exponentially. I worked for the Sports Club Company L.A. as a personal trainer, and exercise instructor, and was soon promoted to member service specialist and sales. From this experience, I realized I had a genuine knack for not only signing up but keeping people accountable, and loved helping patrons find the time to create a healthy lifestyle.

Once the Paseo Club opened, I became the fitness director with responsibility for managing trainers, group X, aquatics, and youth programs.

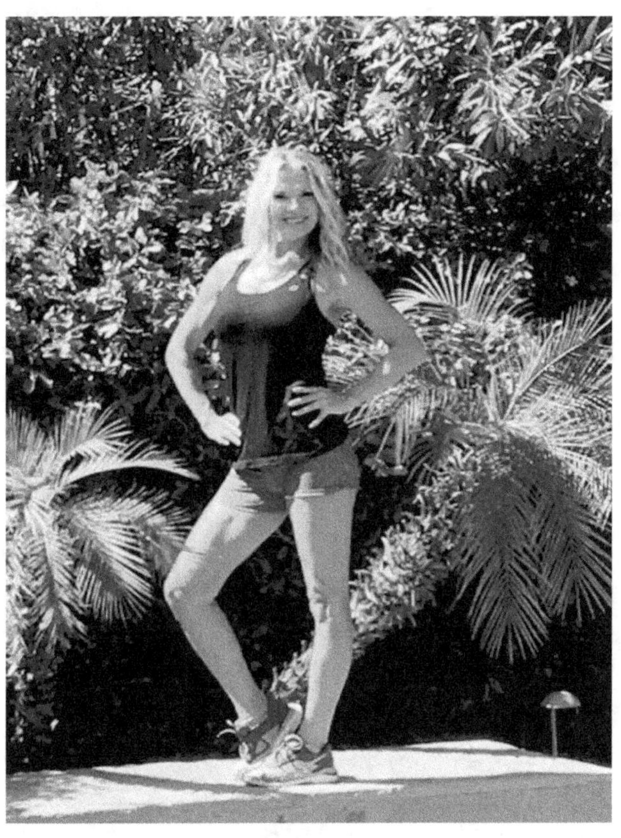

Jodi Stokes, ACE Fitness Certified, Aquatic and Exercise Association (AEA)

As I ran the gym and other departments, I also decided to begin a Boot Camp and Triathlon Club, which became a huge draw for the community. I could go on all day about the Summer Camp, Jodi's Backyard Bootcamp, Flo Jod Run Club, and training hundreds of people to run their first race or half-marathon. For my efforts, I was awarded Elite Trainer and Business Woman of the Year in both 2011 and 2012.

I pride myself on my community involvement and joined Soroptimist International, an international group geared toward helping women. I created and chaired two High-Heel-a-Thons to stomp out domestic violence. I received national acclaim from the Senate, and local acclaim from our Chamber of Commerce, and have since involved myself in many women's organizations.

All of the positions I have held, along with my continued community involvement, buoyed me as I moved back to Scottsdale to open *Goddess Fit* women's gym. The opportunity to support a safe and nonintimidating environment for women to work out was a blessing.

My tenacity and hard work has brought me today to Jodi Stokes Fitness, where I am able to go mobile as a concierge fitness professional and help people to work out in their homes and pools.

Jodi Books-Stokes

I also offer my services to LifeScape Premier concierge medical services. I have recently been honored by *So Scottsdale* magazine among their People to Watch in 2017 and also as a "Trailblazer" 2019 by *Voyage Phoenix* magazine.

I will continue my life's mission to help people live heathy lives and to contribute time to my community.

Thank you for being a part of my journey and life's work.

—Jodi

AUTHOR NOTES

Starting Your Program

The warm-up phase of your program is very important in preparing you both physically and mentally for more strenuous activity to follow. Begin with exercises that call your largest muscles into action. This will raise your body's core temperature and gradually increase the demand placed on your heart. Include exercises that stretch the muscles and move the joints through their full range-of-motion. Five to ten minutes of warm-up will sufficiently increase the blood flow to your muscles, elevate your heart rate, and increase oxygen intake. Always include and prepare your body for warm-up in your exercise program.

Cardio-Respiratory Fitness

Cardio-respiratory fitness is the functional ability of the circulatory system and the respiratory system to deliver oxygen to the muscles and to remove waste products. Fitness researchers have given us precise guidelines for developing and maintaining optimum cardio-respiratory fitness. Cardio-respiratory fitness can be improved by training at least three times a week with a working heart rate elevated between sixty and eighty percent of maximum; and maintained by continuous workload for at least twenty minutes each training session.

Muscular Strength and Endurance

With water exercises, the muscular strength and endurance phase can be combined with the cardio-respiratory phase. The natural resistance of water combined with the increased intensity produces the necessary overload for muscular development. As you use increased effort to overcome the resistance of water, you simultaneously tone and strengthen muscles while conditioning your heart and lungs.

How to Breathe

Breathing correctly, requires you to use the diaphragm. Using the diaphragm gives you seven times the amount of oxygen than shallow chest breathing. I encourage you to exhale during the exertion portion of the exercise—the strenuous portion—and inhale during the preparation of the exercises. Correct breathing will help you to keep your core strong, which will affect the strength of the abdominal area. All fitness levels benefit from healthful centered breathing.

Cool-Down

This phase of your program is designed to decrease body temperature and heart rate, and relax the muscles. This is an excellent time for quiet reflection on slow rhythmic movement. Enjoy the soothing nature of the water.

Sun Care Information

It is important to apply sunscreen thirty minutes before sun exposure, as this will allow the product to dry effectively. You want the sunscreen to bond to the skin so once you begin to perspire it will not sweat off. I recommend a 50 SPF for your face and upper body, and a minimum of 15 SPF properly applied—using one to two milliliters—to the lower body. I also recommend a broad-brimmed hat, sunglasses, and a rash guard, if applicable. Please seek shelter from the sun if feeling too hot or experiencing any skin irritations.

Physician's Referral

Water Exercise by Jodi urges all participants to obtain a physical examination prior to the attendance of any exercise program. In recognition of the possible dangers connected with any physical activity, participants hereby and voluntarily waive any right or cause of action from which any liability may or could accrue to Jodi Books-Stokes. If you have *any* health concerns, please have someone present during your water participation.

WATER EXERCISES

Durations, Body Targets, and Step-by-Step Exercises

Here we go!

FLUTTER KICK, ON THE STEP

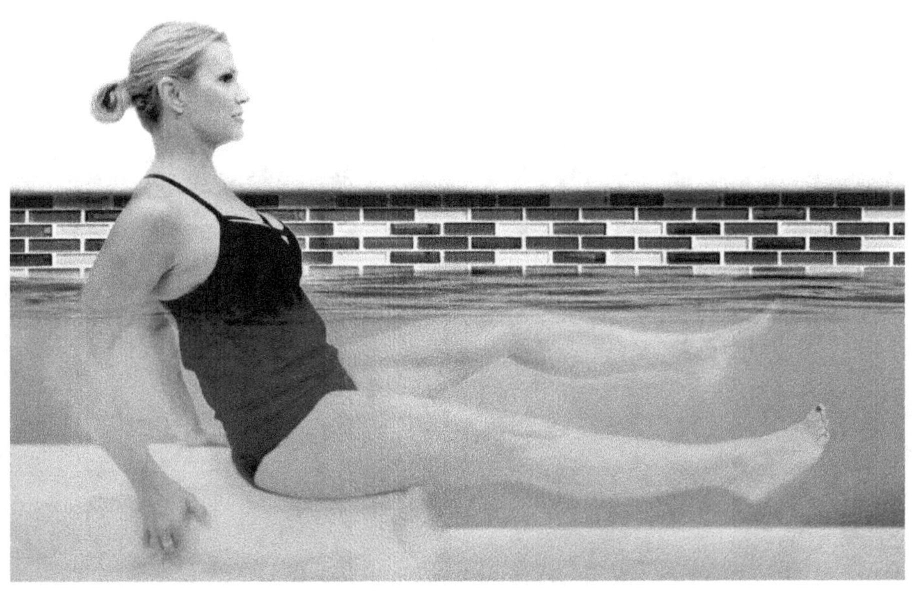

Duration

- 1 minute (beginner 30 seconds)

Targets

- Inner thighs (adductors)
- Outer thighs (abductors)
- Quadriceps
- Core

Exercise

- Lift legs out straight and kick.
- Keep legs under the water.

SCISSOR KICK

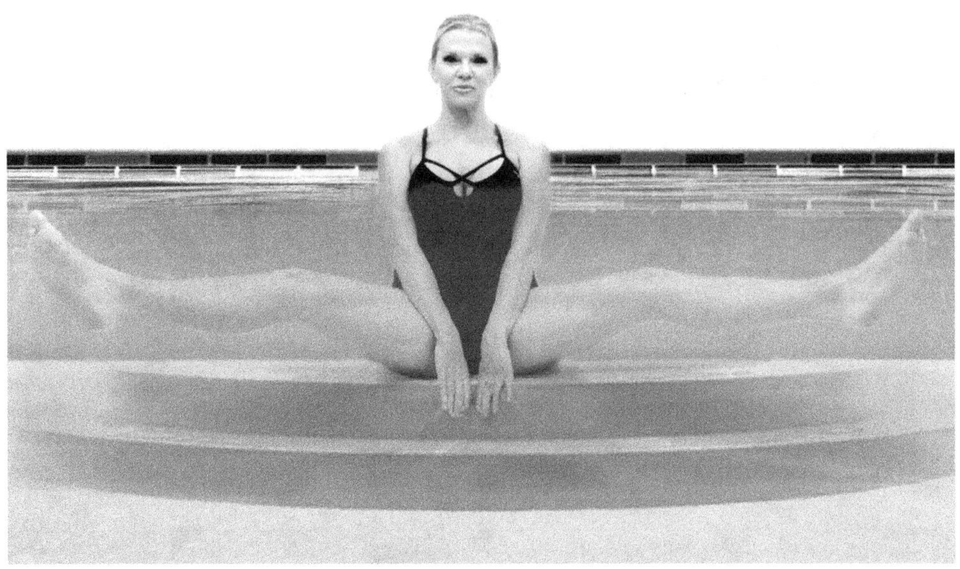

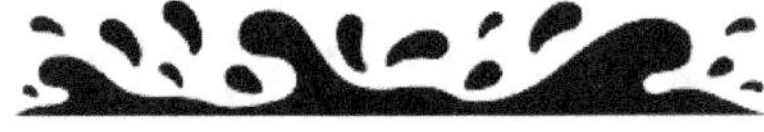

Duration

- Open/close 20 times

Targets

- Inner thighs (adductors)
- Outer thighs (abductors)
- Core

Exercise

- Position body in an "L" shape.
- Open legs.
- Cross legs as you return to a closed position.

FLUTTER KICK, PRONE

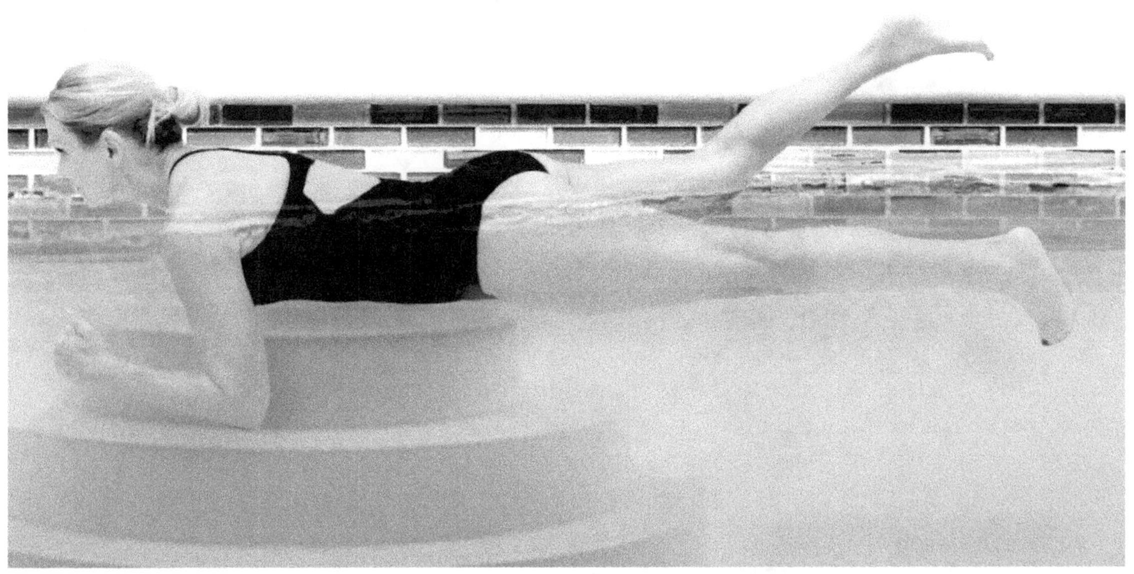

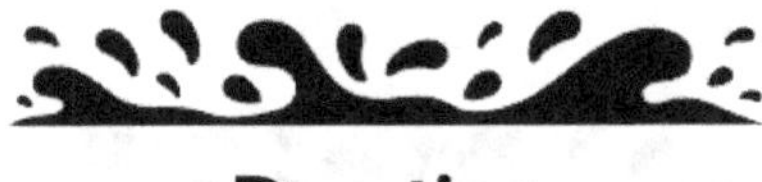

Duration

- 1 minute

Targets

- Glutes
- Quads
- Core

Exercise

- Hands on step, shoulders above hands.
- Kick feet like flippers under water's surface.

BICYCLE KICK

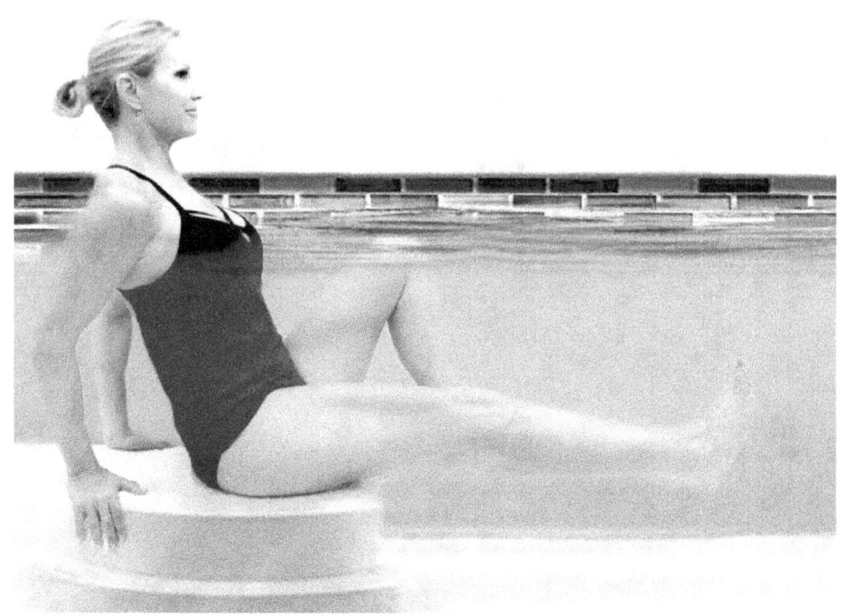

Duration

- 1 minute, each position

Targets

- Quads
- Hamstrings
- Calves
- Core

Exercise

- Sit on edge of step.
- Hands clasp end of step.
- Rotate legs in a bicycle position.
- Sit off the step and maintain core by staying in a seated position.

ABDOMINAL WORK, ON THE STEP

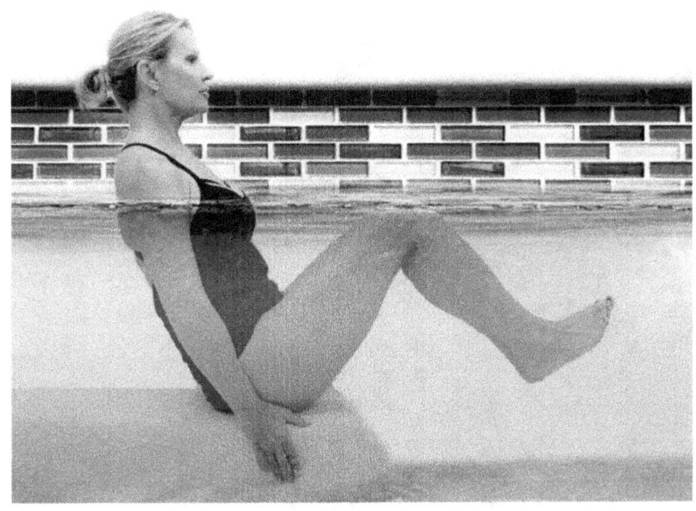

Duration

- 1 minute

Targets

- Core
- Also engages arms and legs

Exercise

- Hands on the edge of step.
- Lift buttocks off of step and bring both knees to chest.

KNEES SIDE TO SIDE

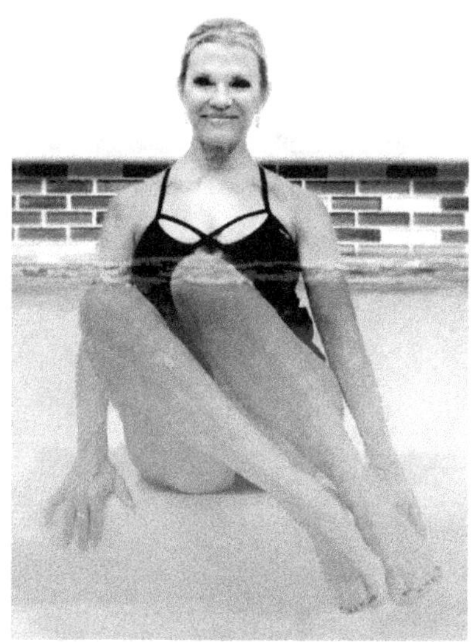

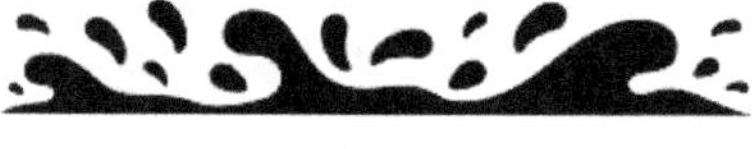

Duration

- 1 minute

Targets

- Abdominals
- Obliques

Exercise

- Hands on edge of step.
- Lift buttocks off the step.
- Straighten legs in front of you.
- Knees to the right.
- Straighten legs.
- Knees to the left.

TOP TO BOTTOM

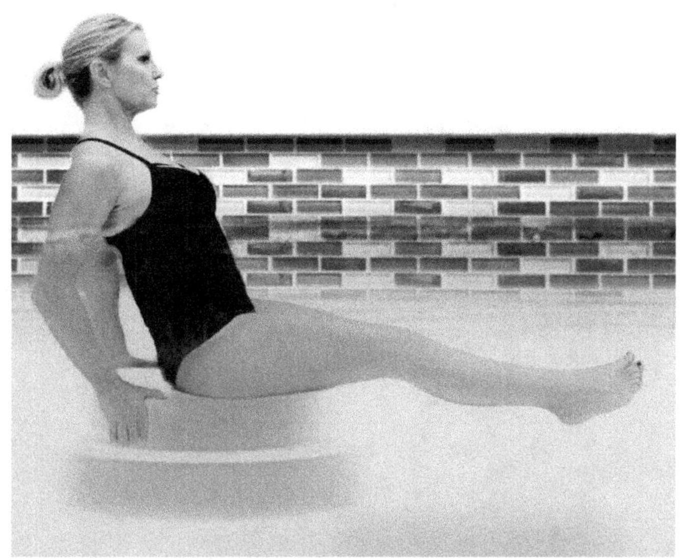

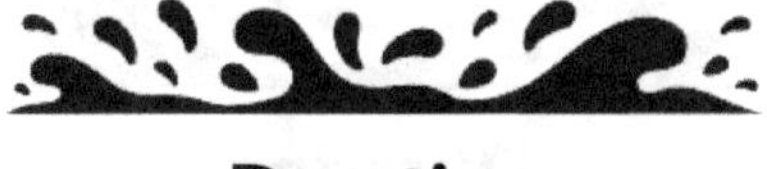

Duration

- 1 minute

Targets

- Lower abdominal

Exercise

- Sit on edge of step.
- Straighten legs toward the surface of the water.
- Drop legs toward the bottom of the pool with flexed feet.

STANDING IN CHEST DEEP WATER

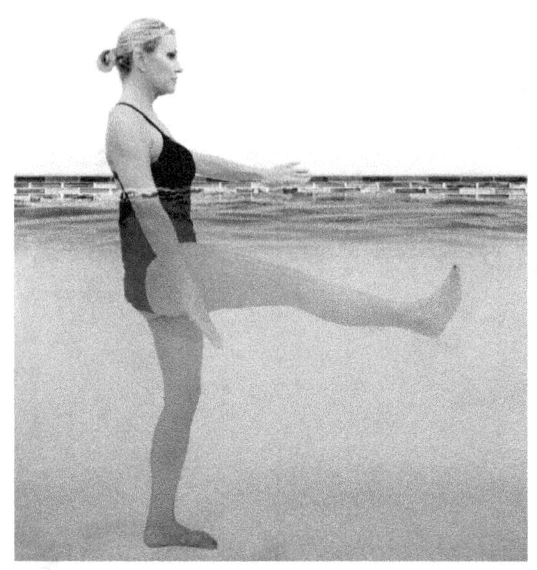

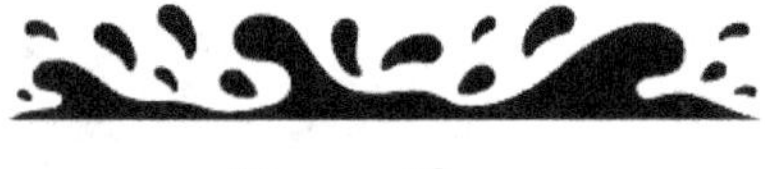

Duration

- 1 minute, each side

Targets

- Quads
- Inner/outer thighs
- Core

Exercise

- Place right hand on the ledge.
- Extend left leg out straight and back down to standing position.
- Turn around and place left hand on ledge.
- Extend right leg out straight and down.

BACKWARD KICK

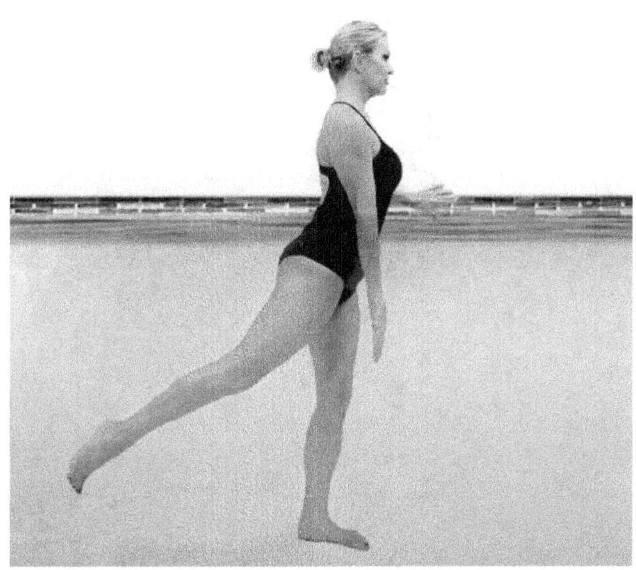

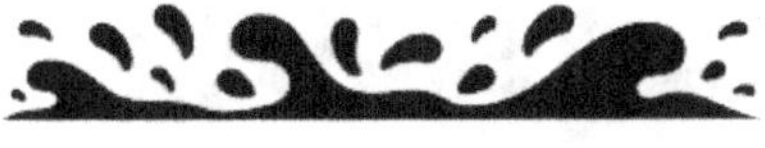

Duration

- 1 minute, each side

Targets

- Hamstrings
- Glutes

Exercise

- Place right hand on ledge.
- Extend left leg back straight and down.
- Turn around and place left hand on ledge.
- Extend right leg back straight and down.

SIDE LATERAL RAISE

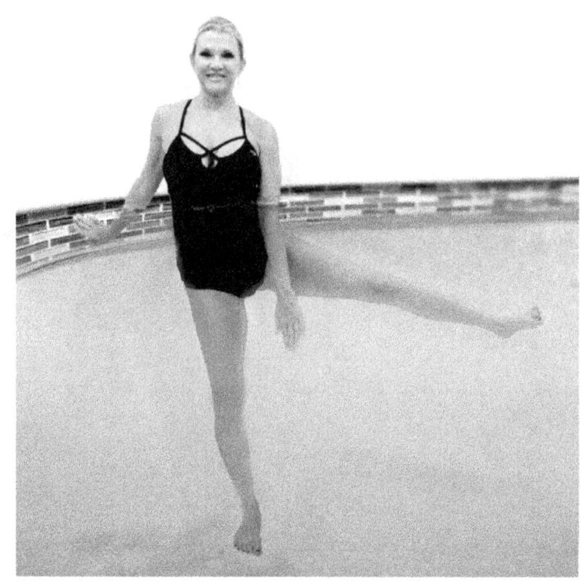

Duration

- 1 minute, each side

Targets

- Outer/inner thighs

Exercise

- Place right hand on ledge.
- Extend left leg out straight to side, lift leg up and down.
- Place left hand on ledge.
- Extend right leg out straight to side, lift leg up and down.

LEG EXTENSION

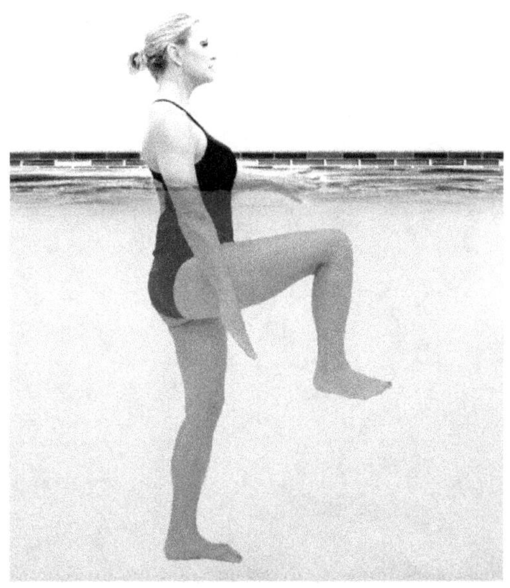

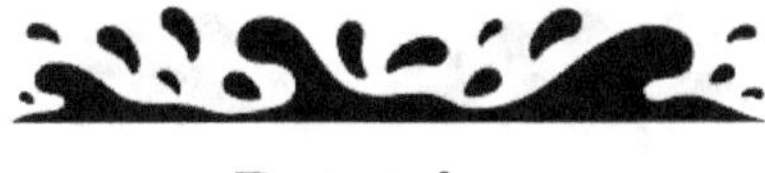

Duration

- 1 minute, each side

Targets

- Quads
- Hamstrings

Exercise

- Place right hand on the ledge.
- Bring left knee up and keep bent.
- Extend leg out straight and back to bent.
- Place left hand on the ledge.
- Bring right knee up and keep bent.
- Extend leg out straight and back to bent.

LEG CURLS

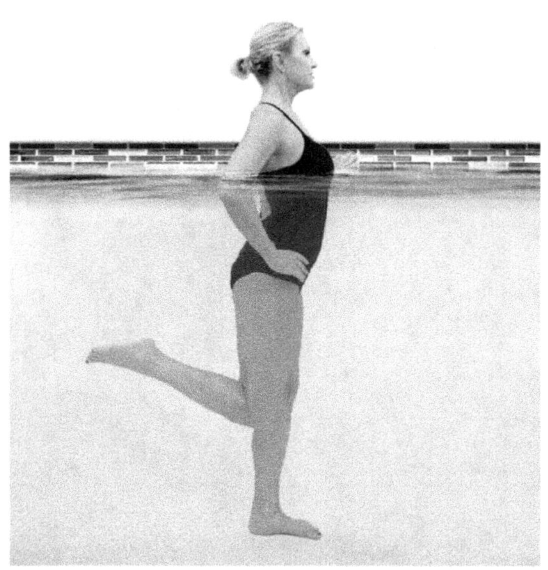

Duration

- 1 minute

Targets

- Hamstring
- Quads

Exercise

- Place right hand on ledge.
- Start with feet together and, with a flexed foot, pull the foot toward your buttocks.
- Place left hand on ledge.
- Start with feet together and, with a flexed foot, pull the foot toward your buttocks.

WATER WALKING/RUNNING

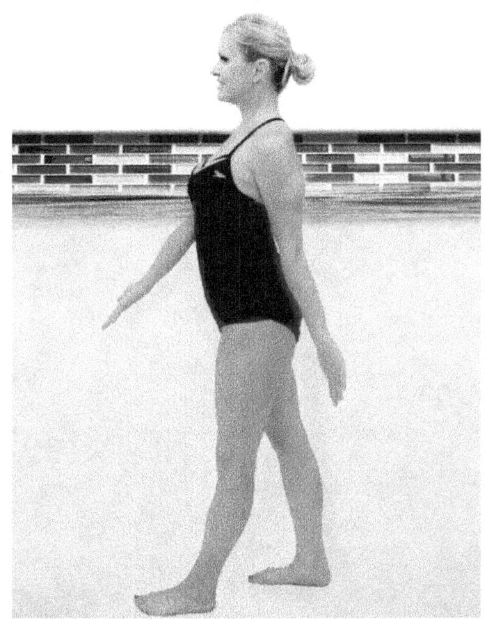

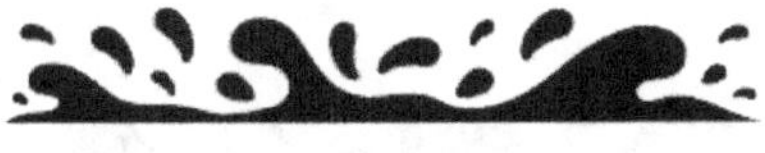

Duration

- One length of the pool and back.

Targets

- Full body

Exercise

- Measure your depth at approximately chest deep so as not to be too buoyant.
- Walk/run in a straight line to the opposite end of the pool and back.
- Arms work in opposition of legs.

STEP TOGETHER STEP

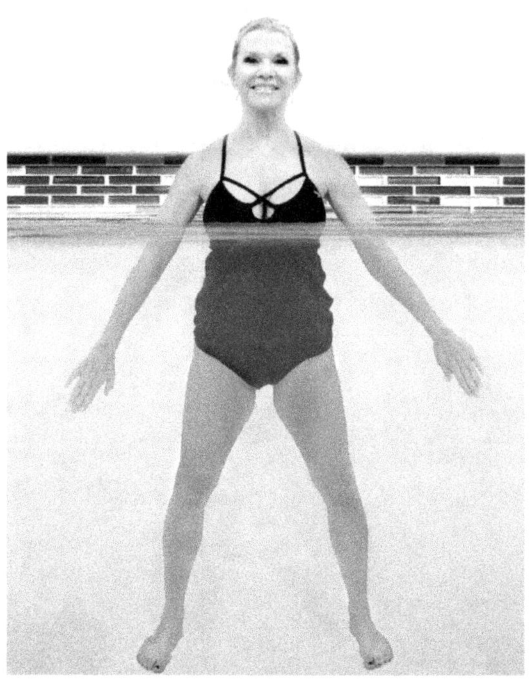

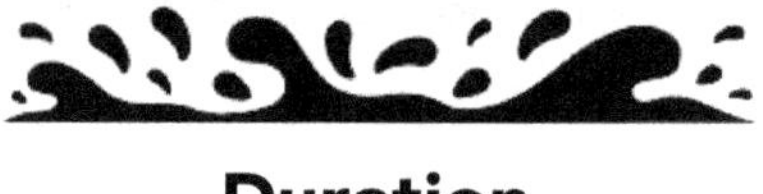

Duration

- 4 steps each way

Targets

- Full body

Exercise

- Begin with legs together.
- Step right 4 times.
- Step left 4 times.
- Hands "scull" (create resistance) outward when you step out and inward when you step together.

CRAB WALKS

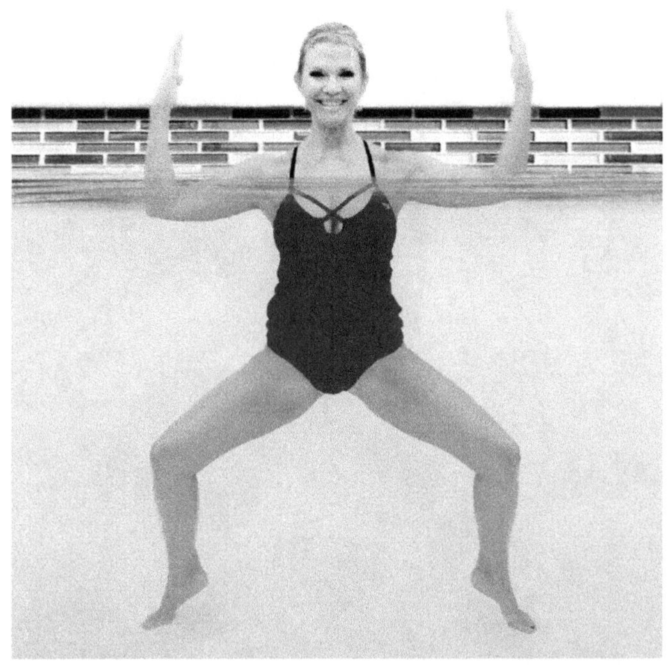

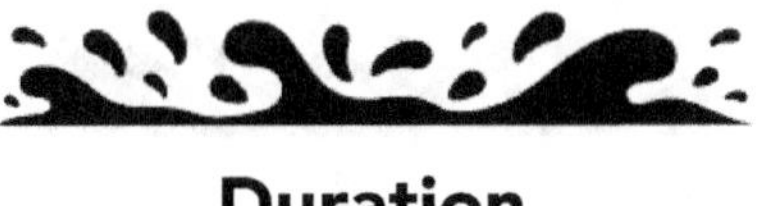

Duration

- 1 minute

Targets

- Full body

Exercise

- Begin on toes with legs in an open position with knees above ankles.
- Tap toes without changing the angle of legs.
- Move across the pool.

TWISTS

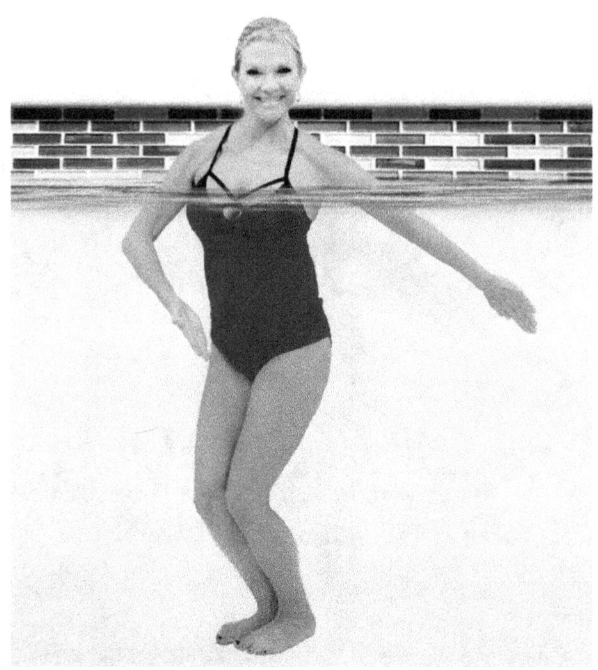

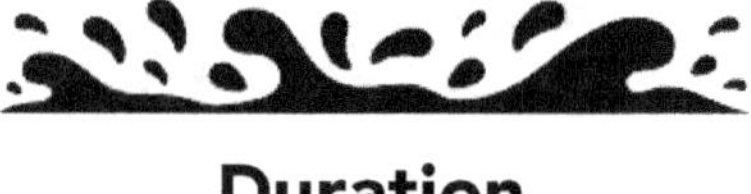

Duration

- 1 minute

Targets

- Full body

Exercise

- Begin with feet and knees together.
- Twist from right to left.
- When knees are right, scull hands left.
- When knees are left, scull hands right.

HIGH KICKS

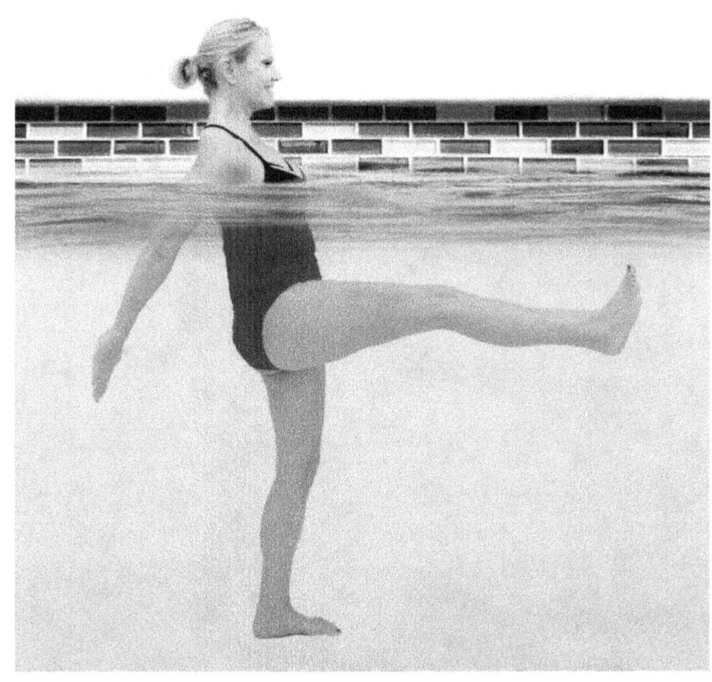

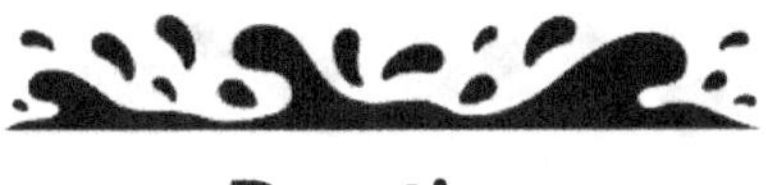

Duration

- 1 minute

Targets

- Full body

Exercise

- Begin standing.
- Extend right leg straight, then left leg.
- Continue switching legs, and do so quickly as to add a hop in the switch.
- Hands scull back and forth in opposition.

PENDULUM KICKS

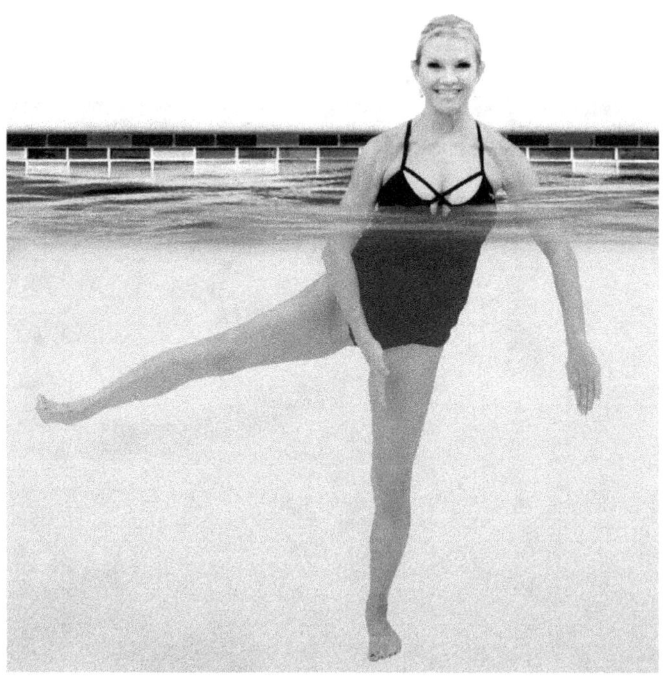

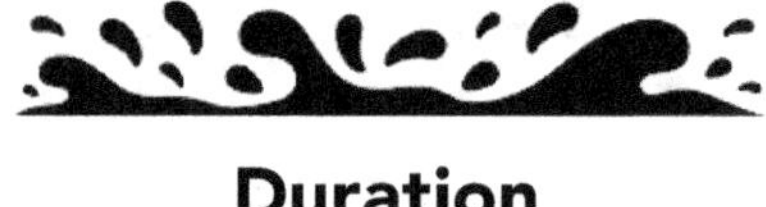

Duration

- 1 minute

Targets

- Full body

Exercise

- Begin standing.
- Extend right leg sideways toward the surface of the water.
- As the right leg comes down, extend left leg toward the surface.
- Hands work in opposition of legs.

QUICK-CHANGE BACK KICKS

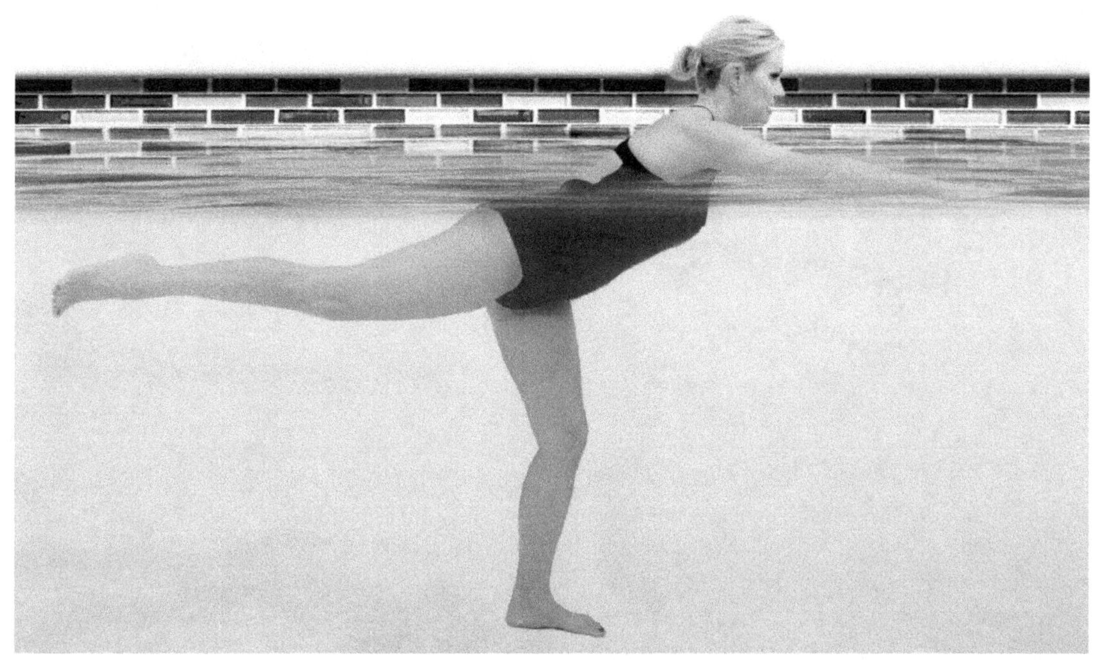

Duration

- 1 minute

Targets

- Full body

Exercise

- Begin standing.
- Extend right leg behind and toward the surface of the water.
- Quick change to the left leg.
- Arms work in opposition.

DEEP-WATER EXERCISES

Durations, Body Targets, and Step-by-Step Exercises

Let's keep going!

34

HIGH KNEE RUNNING

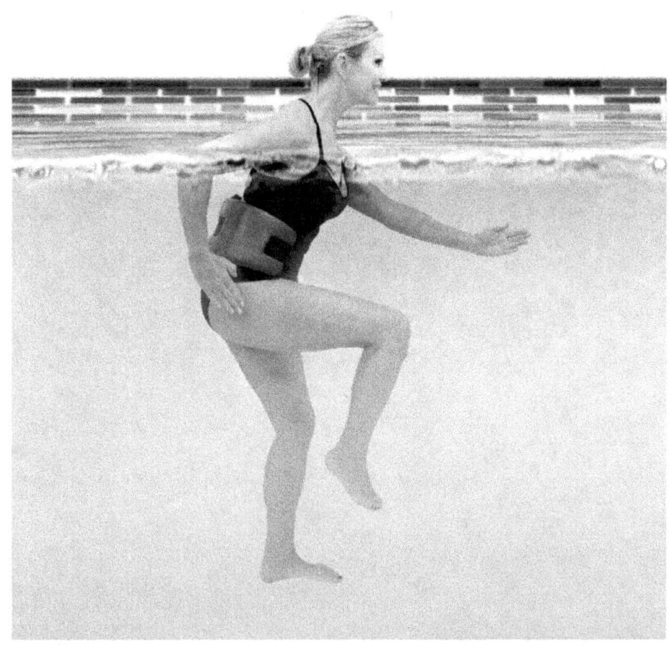

For deep-water exercise, please use a flotation belt,
a pool noodle, or water-specific hand buoys.

Duration

- 1 minute

Targets

- Full body

Exercise

- Begin with the right knee bent while left leg is extended down.
- Switch legs fast as if to simulate running on land.
- Arms work in opposition.

STRADDLE RUN

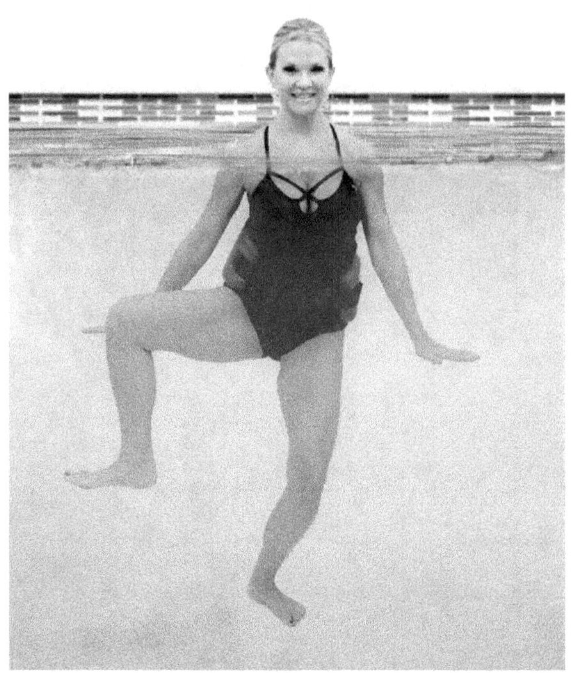

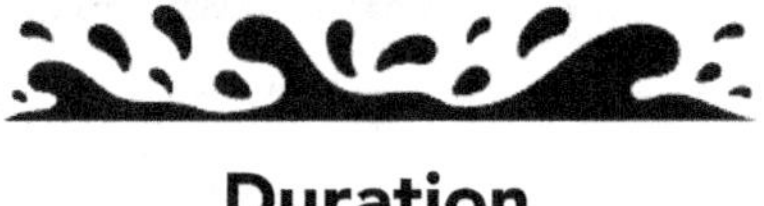

Duration

- 1 minute

Targets

- Full body

Exercise

- Open legs into a straddle position.
- Alternate right knee up and left knee up.
- Arms work in a sculling motion.

OVER-STRIDING

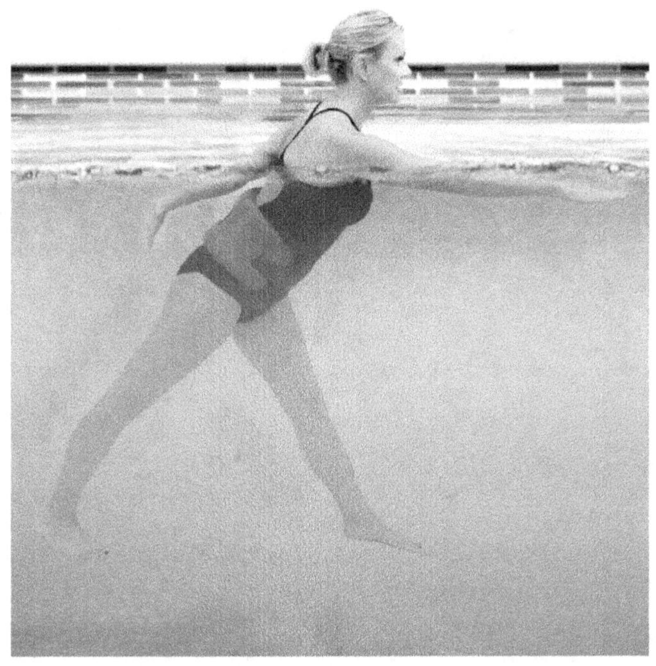

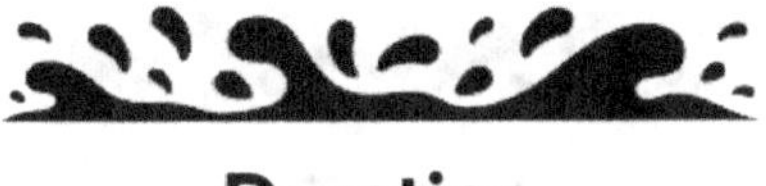

Duration

- 1 minute

Targets

- Full body

Exercise

- Legs perform a swinging motion from front to back, similar to cross-country skiing.

JUMPING JACKS

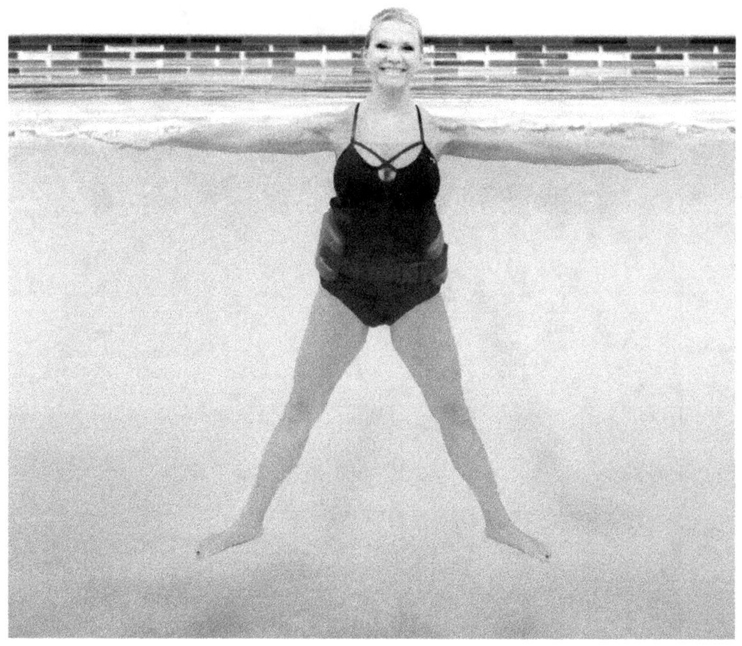

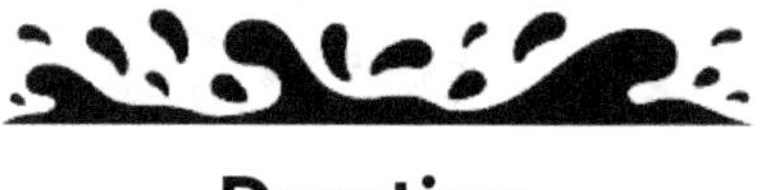

Duration

- 1 minute

Targets

- Full body

Exercise

- Arms and legs are straight down.
- Open arms and legs simultaneously.

FRONT TO BACK ABDOMINALS

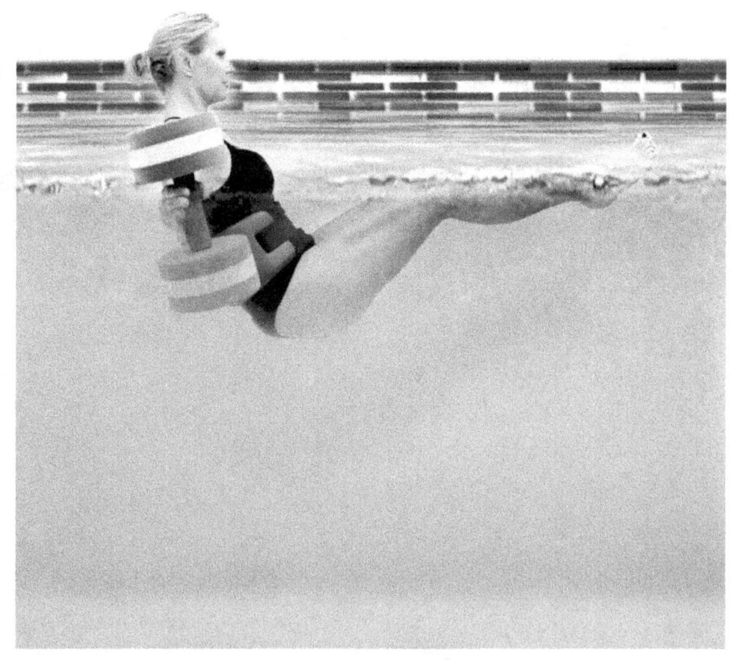

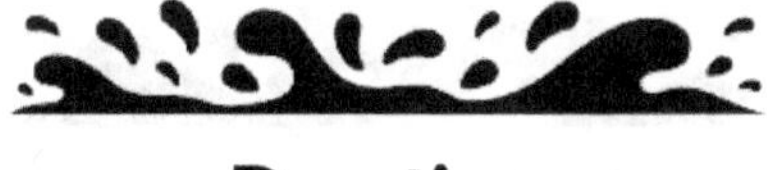

Duration

- 1 minute

Targets

- Core
- Arms

Exercise

- Lay on back (floating).
- Bring knees under your body and roll to your front (prone).
- Bring knees to chest and roll onto back.
- Use arms to help propel the motion forward and backward.

KNEES SIDE-TO-SIDE

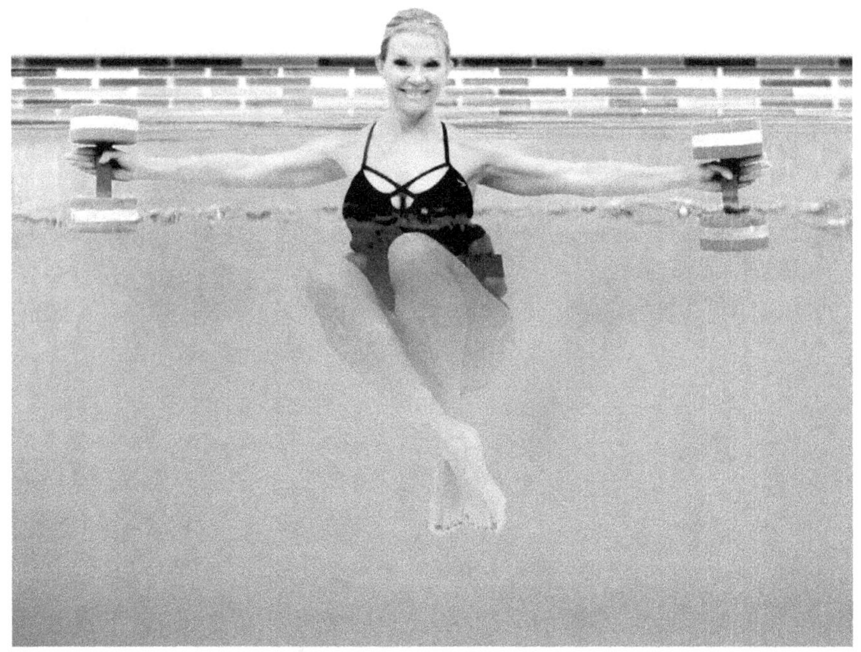

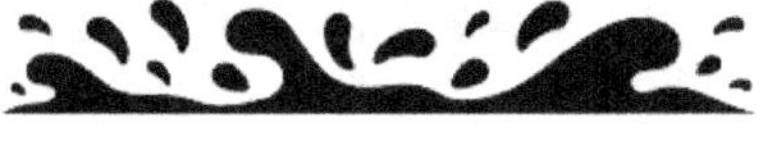

Duration

- 1 minute

Targets

- Core

Exercise

- Bring knees to chest.
- Move them from right to left close to the surface of the water.
- Arms scull forward and back to help buoyancy.

BICYCLE KICK

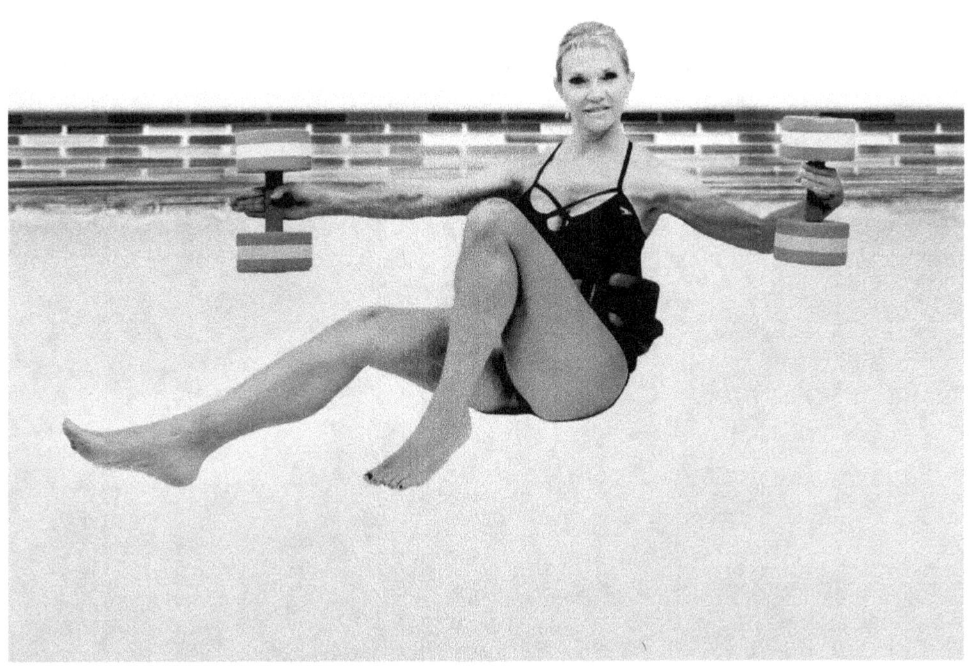

Duration

- 1 minute

Targets

- Core

Exercise

- Bring knees to chest.
- Move knees from left to right while rotating legs in a bicycle motion.

UPPER BODY IN CHEST

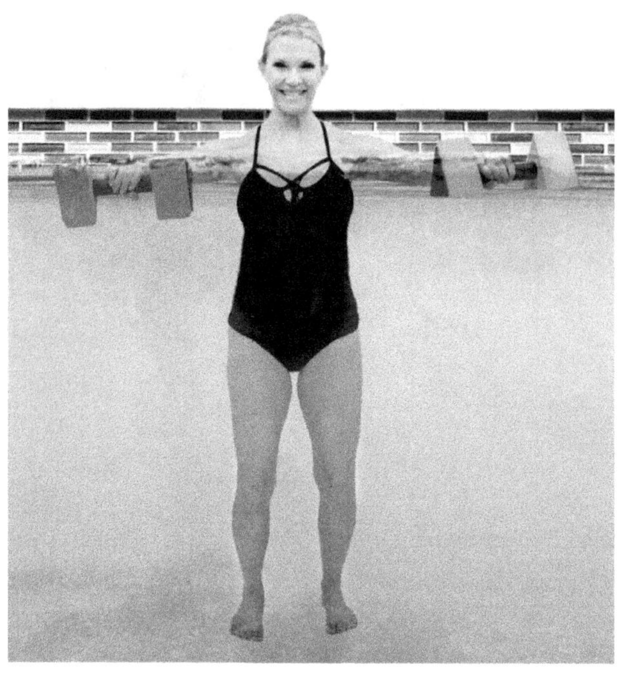

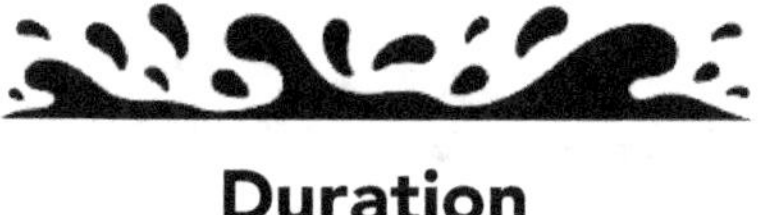

Duration

- 1 minute

Targets

- Chest
- Back
- Triceps
- Balance

Exercise

- Find balance with legs apart while holding the pool noodle just under the surface of the water.
- Push the noodle forward and pull the noodle back.

TRICEPS EXTENSION/BICEPS CURL

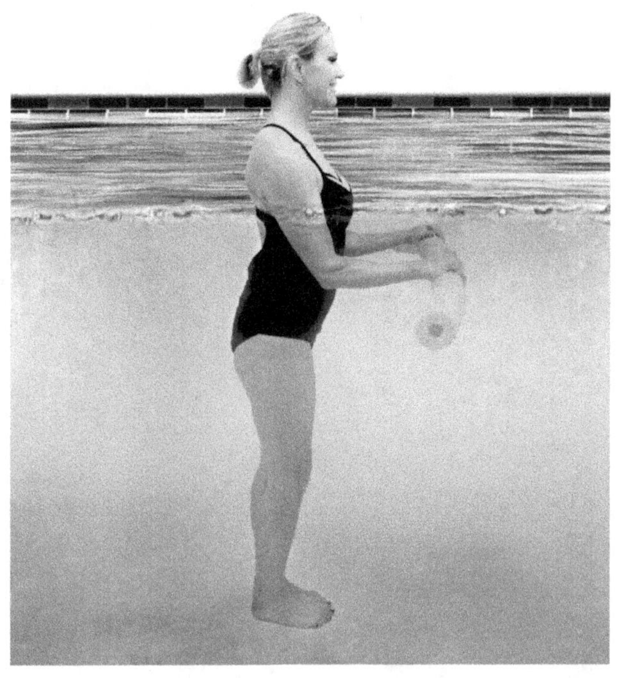

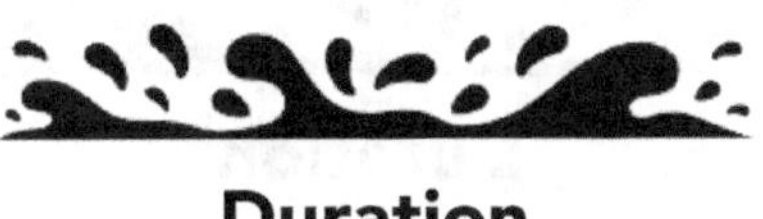

Duration

- 1 minute

Targets

- Triceps
- Biceps

Exercises

Triceps extension

- With arms at 90º (bent elbows), press the noodle to straight arms.
- The noodle will float back to 90º.

Biceps curl

- Turn hands with palms up.
- Repeat the same motion.

STRETCHING

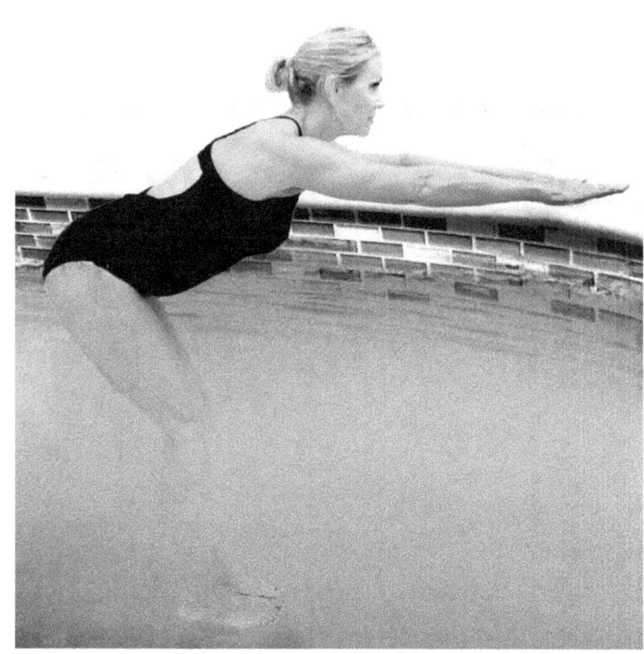

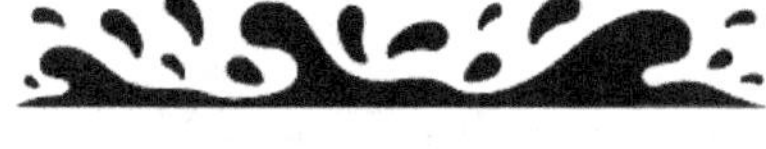

Duration

- 1 minute

Targets

- Specific muscles

Exercises

L-Stretch

- In shallow water, place hands on deck, feet under hips, and press hips back.

Knee to Chest

- Hold knee to chest and ledge with hand.

Wave Press

- Hands together, press from right to left in the water and make a wave.

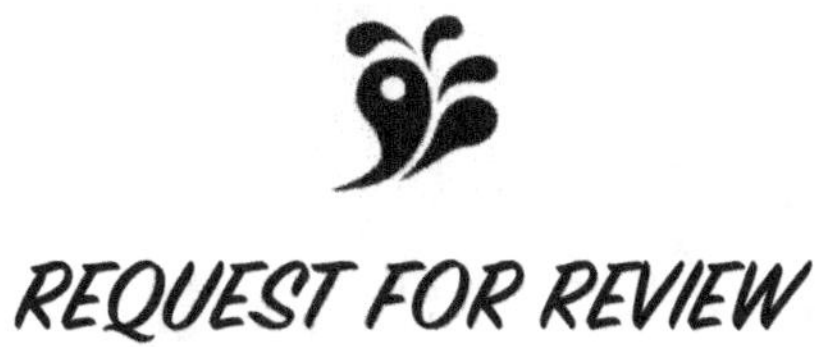

REQUEST FOR REVIEW

If you enjoyed this book, please consider writing a review for it on Jodi Books-Stokes' book page at Amazon.com.

ABOUT THE AUTHOR

Please refer to the Introduction page for details about Jodi Books-Stokes.

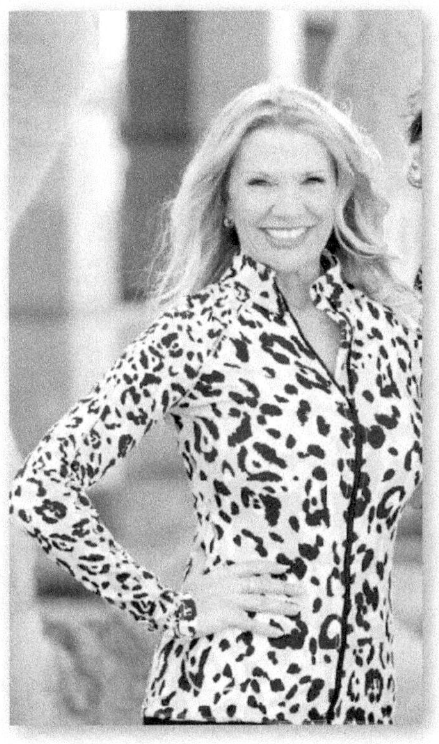